Keto Diet Cookbook For Beginners

Easy Recipes For Fast Weight Loss

I0414805

Eloise Richards

Keto Diet Cookbook For Beginners

ELOISE RICHARDS

Contents:

ELOISE RICHARDS

Keto Diet Cookbook For Beginners
Easy Recipes For Fast Weight Loss

INTRODUCTION

I want to thank you for choosing this book "Keto Diet Cookbook for Beginners: Easy Recipes for Fast Weight Loss".

The modern-day diet and lifestyle are incredibly different from the healthy one that was followed by our ancestors. They suffered from fewer diseases and led long and healthy lives. The rates of modern diseases like obesity and type 2 diabetes were just a fraction of what they are now. These days, people lead a very unhealthy lifestyle and consume too many processed, unhealthy foods. Most people struggle with weight issues and fail to lose extra weight even when they try. Hence, they are all looking for a solution that will show real results. Commonly known as the keto diet, the ketogenic diet has become very popular as of late and is followed by people around the globe. This book will help you understand what the diet is and why people choose to follow it.

Some of you might think that this is just another fad diet that won't work. However, that is far from the truth. This is one of those rare diets that don't require you to fast or starve yourself, go on liquids, or eat tiny, unsatisfying portions. The best part is there is no calorie counting required either. The only prerequisite for the keto diet is that you make a significant reduction in the number of carbohydrates in your diet while you increase the consumption of fats. This might seem unnatural for people who want a diet to lose weight. You might wonder how you will lose fat when you eat more fat. However, this is precisely what the keto diet will help you do.

As you read on, you will understand how this works. You will also get a basic idea of the many ways in which the keto diet can benefit your health and overall well-being. This book will help you understand ketosis, the keto diet, and how you can make it work for you. The recipes in the book will help you get a head start if you decide to follow the keto lifestyle. You will notice that you get to eat a lot of delicious food, even while you lose weight and get healthier. So, if you are ready, let's get started.

Why '***Keto***'?

In many ways, I can honestly say that this is the book that I wish I had been able to access when I started out. I hope you are as excited as I was when I first to embarked on my ketogenic lifestyle. That was in 2016, and I haven't looked back. As cliche as it might sound, I was miserably overweight and inevitably, unhappy. Perhaps like many other folks out there, I had tried every diet you can name and nothing worked. I was even exercising properly! That's when I knew I had to take action, and fast. There was no two ways about it. Either I lose weight and start to live healthily or my quality of life would deteriorate further and beyond repair. For a while, I was doing fine with traditional strategies - namely cutting out foods that I loved while pushing my body to its absolute limit with endless cardio sessions. That lasted six months and around Christmas time, my body's natural tendencies caught up with me. I knew that I had no chance in beating my cravings. So, I visited a nutritionist - something I had put off for years and years but her advice changed my life and it is going to transform yours too! She told me to look into keto-dieting and when I asked what it was, she put it to me this way:

'Keto is the diet that changes you into a fat burner'.

What did she mean by this? In today's world, we are surrounded by high sugar, high carb snacks and fast food. The fats we eat are saturated and not the natural kind found in lean meats, nuts and fruit. From candy bars to easy fries and burgers, our bodies have become used to burning through sugar like it's paper. What the keto lifestyle does however is rewires your metabolism into burning fat the right way. To do this, we readjust our nutritional intake, that is, the food we eat. So what does keto involve exactly?

To put it into simple terms, your diet needs to be centred around:

- High Fat (unsaturated) - 80-150 g
- Medium/Adequate Protein (lean) - 80 - 150 g
- Low Carbohydrate - no more than 60 g

This is the keto motto and the three rules you must live by. Follow them, even vaguely and you will see a difference in your livelihood. However, for the best results, it's important to have meal plans in place as well as a deeper understanding of what foods are good and bad for keto success. In the next chapter, we will be looking at what a keto kitchen looks like and what ingredients make for a tastier and healthier mealtime. Before we get into that, you should be aware that there are three kinds of ketogenic diet.

1. **SKD** (standardized ketogenic dieting)

This is the kind of keto that this book focuses on since it is the easiest to maintain long term and doesn't involve rigid timing, excessive pre-planning and a stressful way of eating.

2. **CKD** (cyclical ketogenic dieting)

Cyclic/cyclical keto is a form of ketogenic diet that involves ratios and distributing what you eat on certain days. One popular form of CKD is where you eat a high carb diet for three days in a week and then for the next two days, you eat no carbs and high protein. While this works for some people, I'm pretty sure you simply don't have the time to be structuring dieting like that. Besides, it often doesn't work long term since we are aiming for a sustainable diet and in effect, a sustainable lifestyle that will keep the pounds off and improve health.

3. **TKD** (targeted ketogenic dieting)

Finally, we have targeted keto dieting. This diet works for those who workout on a consistent basis. With targeted keto, your diet varies depending on when you workout and for how long. You essentially modify your carb intake around the duration of your exercise routine. Again, I would not particularly recommend this one to everyone because it does not enable you to ween off of carbs in a durable way.

- -

In essence, SKD (standardized ketogenic dieting) is our goal and to achieve it, we need to ensure that every meal and snack keeps the high-fat, low carb ratio that leads to mind blowing results. If you need more convincing about keto, here are some of the key health benefits to the diet:

-Lower risk of heart disease.

-Lower cholesterol levels.

-Reduced risk of some forms of cancer.

-Prevents the onset of Alzheimer's disease and dementia.

-Decreases epilepsy in children.

-Lower risk of Parkinson's disease.

-Lower levels of insulin.

-Rejuvenation of skin.

-Prevention of type 2 Diabetes.

Ketosis?

So what is ketosis? Ketosis is a metabolic state in the body where fats are burned for energy. This ketosis is induced when the body does not have enough carbohydrates to meet its energy requirements. The natural tendency of any human body is to burn carbs first to provide energy. When the carbohydrate consumption is reduced in the keto diet, the body turns toward fats. It will burn the fat you consume and the fat that is already stored in your body. Carbs provide the easy-to-burn glucose that your body generally uses to gain energy.

When you stop consuming carbohydrates, your body is denied the glucose it needs. This is when it switches to its fat-burning mode. The body shifts to ketosis, and the stored fat is converted to ketones, which are used as fuel by the body. Usually, the body will refrain from burning this fat in the adipose tissues when it undergoes glycolysis. However, under ketosis, the body quickly works on burning this excess fat. This is why other carbohydrate-rich diets cannot help you lose that extra fat, no matter how hard you try.

The increased levels of insulin will block the release of these fats. The keto diet works the opposite way and helps you meet your weight loss goals. Ketosis is how the body adapts to a low carbohydrate environment and allows your body to survive. To induce this state of ketosis, you have to eat the right keto-friendly foods and ensure the proportion recommended for each of the macros. You should be consuming 70 percent fats, 25 percent proteins, and only 5 percent of your diet should be in the form of carbohydrates. The diet can be adjusted to suit personal needs and preferences. For instance, athletes usually increase the number of carbs they consume because they burn it off fast.

The following information will allow you to understand what you should and should not be eating on the ketogenic diet.

Foods You Can Eat on the Keto Diet

Here is a list of foods that you are allowed to eat while on the keto diet:

* Non-starchy vegetables. Eat more of leafy green vegetables. Add some kale, spinach, lettuce, etc. to your grocery list. Also include veggies like cucumber, zucchini, and asparagus. Eat more of the vegetables that grow above the ground and less of what grows below. Having different vegetables allows you to add variety to your meals.

* Protein from grass-fed and pastured animal meat such as beef, poultry, and pork. Eggs should also be sourced from such animals. Meat should be

consumed in a moderate amount because it can contribute too much protein to your body otherwise. This protein can also be converted to glucose by the body, and it can prevent ketosis.

* Healthy fats from ghee, lard, coconut oil, chicken, goose, and butter. Also, eat avocados and cook with olive oil. Fatty fish are a great way to get omega 3 fatty acids. Heavy cream, yogurt, and cheese can be consumed more than usual.

* Drink black tea, black coffee, water, and bone broth. Don't add sugar to your beverages. Any dairy you consume should be full-fat and not a diet or low-fat variant.

* Nuts are allowed, but they should be low in carbs. Have nuts like pecans and macadamia nuts that are high in fat.

Foods to Avoid on the Keto Diet

Here is a list of foods that you should not eat while on the keto diet:

* Cut off processed foods as much as possible. Wholesome natural foods are recommended. Get rid of your stock of candies, sugary cereals, sodas, cookies, etc. A lot of the "healthy" labeled processed foods contain hidden sugars, so avoid those too. Avoid artificial sweeteners like Equal as well.

* Avoid eating too many fruits because they have a lot of natural sugars. Moderate consumption of berries is ok.

* Avoid any starchy foods. This includes starchy vegetables like potatoes. Also, avoid pasta and white rice. Lower your consumption of lentils and beans too.

* Avoid alcohol, especially beer. Wine is more keto-friendly but should be consumed in moderation.

* Avoid margarine, and don't try to substitute it for butter.

* Use these lists to guide you on your next grocery trip. Buy more keto-friendly foods and avoid buying anything that might cause you to compromise the state of ketosis you have been trying to induce.

More Benefits of the Keto Diet

- It allows you to eat until you are satisfied. You don't have to starve yourself or eat small portions to lose weight. The keto diet lets you eat until satiety, so you don't have to exercise control to stay on a diet. Try to avoid overeating if you aim to lose weight but have all of your main meals on time.

- It does not require calorie counting. Most fad diets or other weight-loss diets will require serious calorie counting. This means you have to ensure that you don't cross a particular threshold of calories per day or per meal. This can be a time consuming and limiting exercise. The keto diet allows you to eat freely without using any calorie calculators. The diet advocates against the consumption of foods that are even labeled low-calorie or no-calorie.

- It promotes better heart health. The modern-day diet has taken a toll on the body and can cause serious heart issues. Studies show that the keto diet promotes good heart health, despite the stigma against fats. Healthy fats will increase good cholesterol levels and lower bad cholesterol levels in your body. A high carb diet with trans fats and refined oils is what causes higher levels of bad LDL in your body. This causes blockage in arteries and can lead to heart diseases.

- It helps to increase energy levels and focus. While it might be the opposite during the initial keto-adaptation phase, you will notice that the keto diet enables you to be more focused and feel re-energized. A high carb diet can leave you feeling tired soon after the body breaks down the carbs. This will make you tired and hungry again. This diet will help you be more productive and be able to focus on your work all day long.

- It will also help in reducing unhealthy cravings. A high carb diet with sugar will increase the incidence of untimely cravings. The body takes more time to burn fat, so you will be less likely to eat between meals. The high carb diet will make you feel hungry as soon as the body burns through the meal. Eating sugars and processed foods can cause an imbalance in hormones as well. This is countered by the keto diet.

- It can help in the regulation of triglyceride levels in your body. Low-fat consumption causes higher levels of triglycerides. Increasing fat consumption will allow the triglyceride level to come back to a normal level again.

- It can lower hypertension and the risk of it. A high carb diet causes an increase in blood pressure. This can then lead to the development of hypertension. Hypertension should be treated as soon as possible, because it can cause other health issues when it gets severe.

- It can help in treating irritable bowel syndrome. A diet that is high in carbs is likely to cause digestive problems and also irritable bowel syndrome. The keto diet can ease this problem and reduce the chances of any such condition.

- It helps reduce inflammation in the body. The keto diet can reduce inflammation caused by a high carbohydrate diet. This can help in pain management related to various inflammatory conditions.

- It helps to burn visceral fat, which is usually hard to get rid of. A high carb diet will result in the accumulation of fat in the abdominal region and cause belly fat. The keto diet can help in the reduction of this fat in an effective way.

There are many other benefits of the keto diet that you will learn about if you try the diet yourself.

ESSENTIALS:

Ingredients For Your Keto Kitchen

Before we get to the recipes, it's time to stock up. You need a range of ingredients which will become the staple of your fridge, cupboards and diet. Knowing what to buy when at the supermarket leaves out the guesswork and prevents you from being tempted into old habits. So stay away from the candy and confectionary and make note of the following must-have ingredients for a Keto diet.

1. Filling, Low Carbohydrate, Non-Starchy Vegetables

We're going to dig deeper here, don't worry - I'm not just pointing out the obvious. When you include low carb veggies into your daily diet, you'll notice a change in the way your body works. Immediately, you'll notice how filling these vegetables are and how your portion size reduces quite rapidly. For the first two or three days, you might feel lethargic if you aren't used to incorporating vegetables into your daily eating habits. Stick with it though! Your body is processing these goodies and very soon, you'll learn to love them and so will your body. You'll feel the effects after a week: no headaches, grogginess or generalized fatigue.

You might also notice that your bowl movements become more frequent. This is because non-starchy low-carb vegetables are antioxidants. They act as detoxifiers for your gut and immune system. So, which vegetables should you be putting into your shopping basket? **Ones that are high in vitamin C, K, and D**. Here are some suggestions but you don't need to be adding all of them. Try some and see which ones you like. It's so important when keto-ing that you enjoy everything you eat. We're in this for the long haul, am I right?

Vegetables:

- Kale
- Spinach
- Broccoli
- Cauliflower
- Brussel Sprouts
- Zucchini (*Courgette* for readers of the EU, the UK, NZ and AUS)
- Carrots

Remember that these vegetables are also formidable sources of dietary fibre and so play a pivotal role in keeping your digestive system healthy and in check. Fibre prevents constipation, irritable bowel syndrome and problems of indigestion.

2. Fish

Now, remember that while we are maintaining a

low-carb diet, moderate to high protein is essential too. Proteins help to maintain brain health, muscle health, replenish and rejuvenate cells and keep the organism healthy. Fish and seafood is the perfect source for keto dieters because unlike red meat, we don't get the backlash of bad fats and high iron concentration. A lot of fish is also high in B vitamins, omega 3, potassium and between you and me - it's basically carb free! If you aren't a fan of fish or seafood, you needn't worry just move on to number 3 but for those willing to give it a go, here are some must-try fish based ingredients for the keto diet.

- Salmon
- Squid
- Tuna (be careful with tuna since it can be high in mercury!)
- Shellfish such as mussels

3. Avocados

Okay let's be honest - you saw this one coming. It wouldn't be a keto cookbook without me shoving AVOCADOS into every free line of the page, right? Well while these wholesome fruits have a bad reputation in the media and are associated with the millennial student diet, there is a reason so many people are picking them up these days. They're awfully popular and with good reason too! In fact, I'd go as far as saying they are essential for the keto diet and it's almost impossible to find keto success without them. Why?

1. Very low in carbs (9g per 100g of fruit)
2. High potassium
3. Low cholesterol
4. Loaded with fibre
5. 26% of daily Vitamin K
6. 18-20% of daily Vitamin C
7. Source of Vitamins E, B6 and B5
8. Low in calories

9.0 sodium - good for lowering blood pressure

Need I say more?

- -

4. Lean Chicken

In the past, I've advised people to pick up chicken when keto-ing but unfortunately, they don't pay attention to what kind of chicken they are buying and eating. Lean cuts of chicken and ones that aren't lean could not be further removed. It's like apples and oranges in terms of difference. In essence, you want to be free range corn-fed chicken fillets. That's a mouthful to say but ideally that's the cut you want to buy and in my experience living in both the United States and in the United Kingdom, these are pretty much available at any supermarket and/or butcher. If worse comes to worst, regular chicken fillets will do. As long as you aren't buying pre-cooked or fried chicken, you're one step ahead of the game as far as the keto diet is concerned.

5. Olive Oil

You want to know why the Greeks and general population of the Mediterranean have such great skin, flowing shiny hair and look great for their age? Well the answer is olive oil. They use it in everything. From Morocco to Italy, it's used in every dish and you need to be replacing any form of butter and oil in your house with olive oil. Why? Because olive oil isn't really an oil at all. It's rich in mono-fats, prevents heart disease, cancer, strokes and liver disease. It also possesses hydrating and replenishing qualities for the hair, nails and skin. Yes, this oil is more expensive but at this point, your best bet is to buy a big bottle of 'extra virgin' olive oil and use small amounts in everything you make. Whether it's a salad or you're frying an egg, anything you would use oil or butter for, olive oil is your super hero. It literally is the fountain of youth we kept hearing about in old movies.

6. Nuts and Seeds

High in protein and unsaturated fat, these are your go-to snack from now on. If you have to transition into them by buying coated or salted, fine. However, do try to eat them 'nude'.

Nuts to Try:

- Cashews
- Walnuts
- Chia seeds
- Flaxseeds
- Sesame seeds
- Brazil nuts

You probably noticed that 'peanuts' are not on the list. Sorry, but their health benefits are minimal and they're a food you should save for a treat and should not be eaten as a staple of a quotidian healthy diet.

7. Fruit

Very few food items can be eaten in such copious amounts but I will say sparingly that you can eat pretty much as much fruit as you'd like. However, there are some fruits which are better for keto diets than others. These include:

1. Blackberries
2. Strawberries
3. Blueberries
4. Cranberries
5. Oranges
6. Red apples

7. Bananas

8. Dark Chocolate

There has to be a silver lining somewhere right? Well there is! All I ask is that you replace your current chocolate habits with dark chocolate (preferably a chocolate that has a high Cocoa percentage - upwards of 60%). Dark chocolate is good for heart health, blood pressure and reducing stress.

9. Brown Rice and Brown Pasta

Similar to other carbs, we need to keep this on the down-low but you need ***some*** carbs for a healthy diet. Substitute any carb you'd normally have with the brown alternative. The same applies to breads - opt for wholegrain instead of white.

10. Eggs

A cheap, healthy and easily accessible form of protein which is high in B vitamins and low in calories. You can use eggs instead of other proteins which makes them versatile. Duck, goose or chicken eggs will do.

- -

Needless to say, the rest is down to you as you craft your keto diet. Make sure whatever other foods you pick up, that they're keto-friendly - low carb, moderate protein, high fat. Nonetheless, these ten items should be your go to whenever you enter a store to do your weekly grocery shopping.

Now it's time to get cooking.

COOKBOOK

Ketogenic Breakfast Recipes

Keto Taco Breakfast Skillet

Serves: 3

Ingredients:

- ½ pound ground beef
- 5 large eggs
- 1/3 cup water
- 2 tablespoons heavy cream
- 1 small avocado, peeled, pitted, cubed
- 2 tablespoons sour cream
- 1 green onion, sliced
- ½ jalapeño, sliced (optional)
- 2 tablespoons taco seasoning
- ¾ cup shredded sharp cheddar cheese, divided
- 2 tablespoons sliced black olives
- 1 small tomato, diced
- 2 tablespoons salsa
- 1 handful cilantro, chopped

Directions:

Place an ovenproof skillet over medium-high heat. Add beef and cook until brown. Discard excess fat from the pan.

Add taco seasoning and water into the skillet and mix well. Lower the heat and cook until thick. Turn off the heat.

Meanwhile, whisk eggs in a bowl. Add ½ cup cheddar cheese and cream and whisk well.

Take out half the beef mixture and place in a bowl.

Add egg mixture into the skillet and mix well.

Transfer the skillet into an oven.

Bake in a preheated oven at 375°F for about

25-30 minutes or until cooked.

Spread beef that was set aside. Sprinkle remaining cheddar cheese, tomato, olives, avocado, and green onion on top. Drizzle salsa and sour cream on top.

Sprinkle cilantro and jalapeño and serve.

Huevos Pericos

Serves: 8

Ingredients:

4 teaspoons butter

2 Roma tomatoes, chopped

8 eggs

Pepper to taste

Salt to taste

4 teaspoons olive oil

4 green onions, thinly sliced; keep the white and green parts separate

4 tablespoons milk

Directions:

Place a skillet over medium heat. Add oil and butter. When butter melts, add the whites of the green onion and sauté until translucent.

Add tomatoes and green part of the green onions and cook until slightly dry.

Meanwhile, add milk and eggs in a bowl and whisk them well.

Pour eggs into the pan and stir constantly until the eggs are cooked.

Season with salt and pepper and serve.

Sausage Breakfast Sandwich

Serves: 2

Ingredients:

2 large eggs

4 sausage patties

4 tablespoons sharp cheddar cheese

1 teaspoon sriracha sauce or to taste

¼ teaspoon red pepper flakes (optional)

2 tablespoons cream cheese

Little butter, grease

Directions:

Whisk together eggs, red pepper flakes, salt and pepper in a bowl.

Add cream cheese and sharp cheddar cheese into a microwave-safe bowl. Cook for 20 seconds or until it melts. Add sriracha sauce and stir.

Place a skillet over medium flame. Add a little butter and let it melt.

Pour ½ the beaten egg mixture. Spread half the cheese mixture in the center of the omelet and let it cook for a minute.

Fold the edges of the omelet over the cheese. Carefully slide on to a plate.

Repeat steps 3-5 and make the remaining omelet.

Meanwhile, heat the patties following the instructions on the package.

Place 2 patties on a serving platter. Place one omelet on each patty. Place the remaining 2 patties over the omelet to complete the sandwiches.

Smoky Pulled Pork Breakfast Hash

Serves: 4

Ingredients:

4 tablespoons ghee or butter or coconut oil

1 teaspoon paprika

½ teaspoon garlic powder

6 Brussels sprouts, halved

¼ cup chopped red onion

4 eggs

2 turnips, diced

Salt to taste

Pepper to taste

2 cups chopped lacinato kale

6 ounces pulled pork

Directions:

Place a pan over medium flame. Add oil and once it heated, add turnip, garlic powder, paprika, and pepper and sauté for 3-4 minutes. Stir occasionally.

Stir in Brussels sprouts, onion, and kale and cook until slightly tender.

Stir in the pork and heat thoroughly.

Make 4 cavities at different spots in the mixture, big enough for an egg to fit in.

Break an egg into each cavity. Cover the pan and cook the eggs to the desired doneness.

Serve hot.

Spanish Baked Eggs

Serves: 4

Ingredients:

2 tablespoons olive oil

1 teaspoon paprika

2 tomatoes, sliced

Salt to taste

Pepper to taste

4 ounces manchego cheese, grated

2 chorizo sausages, chopped

½ teaspoon ground cumin

2/3 cup roasted peppers strips

4 eggs

2 teaspoons finely chopped parsley

Directions:

Place a pan on medium flame and heat some oil. When the oil is heated, add chorizo, cumin, and paprika and cook for 4-5 minutes until cooked thoroughly.

Add tomatoes and cook until the tomatoes are mashed. Stir in the roasted pepper, pepper and salt and mix well. Turn off the heat.

Take 4 small baking dishes. Divide the mixture equally into the dishes. Spread it all over the dishes. Make a cavity in the center of each dish, big enough for an egg to fit in.

Break an egg into each cavity. Scatter cheese and parsley on top.

Bake in a preheated oven at 390° F for about 5-10 minutes, depending on the desired doneness.

Serve hot.

Breakfast Bowl

Serves: 2

Ingredients:

14.5 ounces radishes, scrubbed, cubed

½ cup shredded cheddar cheese

½ teaspoon Himalayan pink salt

7 ounces ground sausage

2 large eggs

½ cup shredded cheddar cheese

Pepper to taste

Salt to taste

Directions:

Place an ovenproof skillet over medium heat. Add the sausage to the skillet and cook until they turn brown.

Remove sausage with a and place on a plate.

Add radish into the pan along with salt and pepper and cook until fork tender.

Meanwhile, cook eggs, sunny side up, to the desired doneness.

Divide radishes among 2 bowls. Place sausage over it followed by cheese and eggs.

Serve immediately.

Steak and Eggs

Serves: 2

Ingredients:

2 tablespoons butter

8 ounces sirloin

Pepper to taste

Salt to taste

6 eggs

½ avocado, peeled, pitted sliced

Directions:

Place a skillet over medium heat. Add sirloin and cook until done.

Remove the sirloin and keep it on a cutting board. When it cools down, cut into bite-sized pieces. Sprinkle salt and pepper.

Discard the fat in the skillet.

Add a little butter into the skillet and cook 1-2 eggs at a time, to the desired doneness.

Divide steak among 4 plates. Serve eggs and avocado slices along with steak.

Spicy Baked Eggs with Cheesy Hash

Serves: 6

Ingredients:

10 ounces zucchini, chopped

1 medium red bell pepper, chopped

12 ounces cauliflower, chopped

2 tablespoons coconut oil, melted

2 teaspoons onion powder

2 teaspoons smoked paprika

1 teaspoon garlic powder

1 medium avocado, peeled, pitted, sliced

1 jalapeño, sliced (optional)

4 teaspoons Tajin seasoning

½ cup Mexican blend shredded cheese

6 tablespoons shredded Cotija cheese

6 large eggs

Salt and pepper to taste

Directions:

Place a sheet of foil in a large baking dish.

Place the cauliflower, zucchini and red pepper in the dish. Pour oil on top. Sprinkle onion powder, garlic powder and paprika over the vegetables and toss well. Spread it evenly in the dish.

Bake in a preheated oven at 350°F for 15 minutes.

Remove the dish and sprinkle Mexican cheese all over the vegetables.

Crack the eggs at different spots over the vegetables. Place avocado slices in the gap between the eggs and on the sides.

Place it back in the oven and cook the eggs to the

desired doneness.

Sprinkle Cotija cheese, Tajin seasoning, and jalapeños if using and serve.

Breakfast Burger Fat Bombs

Serves: 10

Ingredients:

½ pound ground beef

Freshly ground pepper to taste

Kosher salt to taste

1 ½ tablespoons cold butter, cut into 10 small cubes

¼ teaspoon garlic powder

10 thinly sliced tomatoes, to serve

4 ounces block cheddar cheese, cut into 10 cubes

Mustard to serve

Lettuce leaves to serve

Cooking spray

Directions:

Grease a mini muffin pan with cooking spray.

Add beef, garlic powder, salt and pepper into a bowl and mix well.

Place a tablespoon of beef mixture in each of 10 muffin cups in the muffin pan.

Press it well onto the bottom of the cup. Place a cube of butter in each.

Place a tablespoon of beef mixture. Press it such that the butter is enclosed between the beef layers.

Place a cube of cheese in each of the 10 cups. Divide the remaining beef mixture among the cups. The cheese cube should be enclosed between the beef layers.

Bake in a preheated oven at 350°F for 10-15 minutes or until brown in color.

Remove from the oven and allow it to cool. Once cool, invert onto a plate.

Place lettuce leaves on a serving platter. Place burgers over it. Place a tomato slice on each burger. Drizzle mustard on top and serve.

Bacon and Spinach Frittata

Serves: 6

Ingredients:

12 duck eggs or 16 hen eggs

8 ounces bacon, cut into ½ inch pieces

4 cups spinach or collard greens

2 rosemary sprigs, finely chopped

2 tablespoons ghee

3 cups green beans, cooked, halved

8 ounces cherry tomatoes, halved (optional)

Salt to taste

Pepper to taste

Directions:

Place an ovenproof skillet over medium flame. Add ghee. When ghee melts, add rosemary and bacon and cook until slightly crisp.

Add spinach, tomato and green beans and cook until slightly tender.

Meanwhile, add eggs into a bowl and whisk well. Pour all over the vegetables in the pan. Cook for 4-5 minutes. Turn off the heat.

Transfer the skillet into a preheated oven.

Bake at 350°F for 5-10 minutes or until set. Remove the skillet from the oven and let it cool for a few minutes.

Cut into 6 equal wedges and serve. To have for lunch or dinner, serve with a keto-friendly salad.

Low-Carb Overnight Mocha Chia Seed Pudding

Serves: 4

Ingredients:

½ cup heavy cream

6 tablespoons chia seeds

3 teaspoons granulated stevia

¼ teaspoon pure almond extract

1/8 teaspoon sea salt

20 almonds, toasted, chopped

1 ½ cups strong brewed coffee

4 tablespoons unsweetened cocoa powder

1 teaspoon vanilla extract

20 cherries, pitted, halved, to garnish

Directions:

Add heavy cream, chia seeds, stevia, almond extract, coffee, cocoa, vanilla extract and salt into a bowl. Stir well.

Cover the bowl with plastic wrap and chill for 7—8 hours.

Transfer into a blender. Blend until smooth.

Divide into 4 glasses. Chill for an hour.

Sprinkle almonds and cherries on top and serve.

Chai Latte

Serves: 4

Ingredients:

2 tablespoons chai tea

1 cup heavy whipping cream

4 cups water

Directions:

Follow the instructions on the package and brew the tea, using 4 cups water. The brewed tea should be boiling hot.

Add cream into a glass bowl and microwave for about 15-20 seconds.

Pour tea into mugs. Pour cream on top and serve.

Frozen Bulletproof Coffee

Serves: 2

Ingredients:

1 ½ cups freshly brewed hot black coffee

2 cups ice cubes

1 banana, sliced, frozen

½ teaspoon ground cinnamon

1/8 teaspoon salt

2 tablespoons solid coconut oil

2 tablespoons peanut butter

2 tablespoons plain protein powder (optional)

½ teaspoon vanilla extract

Directions:

Pour hot coffee into the blender. Add in the oil. Cover partially the blender jar and cover the lid with kitchen towel.

Set the blender on medium-high and blend until creamy and brown. Coconut oil should be emulsified.

Add ice cubes, banana, cinnamon, salt, peanut butter, protein powder and vanilla and blend until creamy.

Pour into 2 glasses and serve.

Liquid Fat Bomb Smoothie

Serves: 4

Ingredients:

2 cups full fat coconut milk

4 egg yolks

1 1/3 cups frozen berries

1 cup water

2 scoops whey protein powder, unsweetened

Directions:

Add coconut milk, yolks, berries, water and protein powder into a blender and blend until it gets frothy.

Pour into 4 glasses and serve with ice if desired.

Peanut Butter Smoothie

Serves: 2

Ingredients:

2 cups coconut milk

2 tablespoon peanut butter

1 teaspoon ground cinnamon

4 tablespoons coconut oil

1 teaspoon vanilla extract

Ice cubes, as required

Directions:

Add coconut milk, peanut butter, cinnamon, coconut oil, vanilla and ice cubes into a blender.

Blend well until it gets smooth.

Pour into 2 glasses and serve.

Bulletproof Coconut Smoothie

Serves: 2

Ingredients:

1 cup coconut milk

2 tablespoons MCT oil or Brain octane oil

4 tablespoons whey protein powder

Stevia drops to taste

½ cup filtered water

1 vanilla bean, scrape the seeds

Zest of a lemon, grated

Directions:

Add coconut milk, MCT oil, protein powder, stevia, water, vanilla bean seeds and lemon zest in a blender.

Blend well until it gets smooth and creamy.

Pour into 2 glasses and serve.

Salted Caramel Cashew Smoothie

Serves: 2

Ingredients:

2 cups cashew milk, unsweetened

Ice cubes, as required

Pumpkin pie spice, to sprinkle

4 tablespoons sugar-free salted caramel syrup

1/3 cup heavy cream

Directions:

Add cashew milk, ice, caramel syrup and heavy cream in a blender.

Blend well until it gets smooth.

Pour into 2 glasses.

Sprinkle pumpkin pie spice on top and serve.

Cinnamon Almond Butter Breakfast Shake

Serves: 2

Ingredients:

3 cups nut milk of your choice, unsweetened

4 tablespoons almond butter

1 teaspoon ground cinnamon

¼ teaspoon almond extract

Ice cubes, as required

2 scoops collagen peptides

4 tablespoons golden flax meal

30 drops stevia

¼ teaspoon salt

Directions:

Add nut milk, almond butter, cinnamon, almond extract, ice cubes, golden flax meal, stevia and salt into a blender.

Blend well until it gets smooth and frothy.

Add collagen peptides and give short pulses until well combined. Do not over blend.

Pour into 2 glasses and serve.

Peanut Butter Chocolate Milkshake

Serves: 2

Ingredients:

2 cups coconut milk, unsweetened

2 tablespoons plain peanut butter, unsweetened

A large pinch sea salt

2 tablespoons cocoa powder, unsweetened

10 drops stevia drops

Directions:

Add coconut milk, peanut butter, salt, cocoa powder and stevia into a blender

Blend well until it gets smooth and frothy.

Pour into smoothie glasses and serve.

Ketogenic Snack Recipes

Zucchini Nacho Chips

Serves: 8

Ingredients:

2 large zucchini, cut into thin round slices

2 tablespoons Tex-Mex seasoning

2 cups coconut oil

Salt to taste

Directions:

Place a colander over a bowl. Place zucchini slices in the colander. Season with salt and mix using your hands. Set aside for 5 minutes.

Press the zucchini slices of excess moisture.

Place a pan over medium flame. Add oil and let it heat.

When the oil reaches 350 ° F, fry few zucchini chips at a time until golden brown.

Remove and place on a plate.

Dust with Tex-Mex seasoning and serve.

Leftovers can be stored in an airtight container until use.

Cheddar Cheese and Bacon Balls

Serves: 14-16 (3-4 balls per serving)

Ingredients:

10-11 ounces bacon

10-11 ounces cheddar cheese

10-11 ounces cream cheese

4 ounces butter, at room temperature, divided

1 teaspoon chili flakes (optional)

1 teaspoon pepper (optional)

Salt to taste

Directions:

Place a pan over medium heat. Add half the butter and melt. Add bacon and cook until crisp. Remove bacon with a slotted spoon and place on paper towels.

When cool enough to handle, crumble the bacon. Set aside in a shallow bowl.

Pour the remaining fat from the pan into a bowl. Add remaining butter, cheddar cheese, cream cheese, chili flakes, pepper and salt and mix well, using your hands.

Chill for 20-30 minutes.

Divide the mixture into 40-50 portions and shape into balls.

Dredge the mixture in bacon and serve.

Store leftovers in an airtight container in the refrigerator.

Tuna Salad Cups

Serves: 4

Ingredients:

2 large eggs, hard boiled, peeled, chopped

3 tablespoons keto-friendly mayonnaise

½ tablespoon lemon juice

1/8 teaspoon lemon zest

1 can tuna (5 ounces) packed in olive oil

Salt to taste

Freshly ground pepper to taste

8 Bibb lettuce leaves

2 strips bacon

1 tablespoon sour cream

½ stalk celery, thinly sliced

1 scallion, sliced

1 small tomato, cut into 4 slices

Directions:

Place a pan over medium flame. Add the bacon and cook until it becomes crisp.

Remove and place on a plate.

When cool enough to handle, cut into bite size pieces.

Add mayonnaise, lemon zest, lemon juice, tuna oil (from can), sour cream, celery, salt and pepper into a bowl and whisk until well combined.

Add most of the scallions, tuna, egg and most of the bacon and fold gently. Taste and adjust the seasoning if required.

Season tomato slices with salt and pepper.

Place the lettuce leaves on a serving platter. Divide the tuna salad mixture among the lettuce leaves. Place a tomato slice in each cup.

Garnish with remaining bacon and scallions and serve.

Black and White Fat Bombs

Serves: 24

Ingredients:

4 cups slivered almonds

3-4 tablespoons swerve or erythritol

2 teaspoons grated orange zest

4 tablespoons unsweetened cocoa powder

2 cups virgin or extra-virgin coconut oil

4 teaspoons vanilla extract

¼ teaspoon kosher salt

Directions:

Take 2 mini muffin tins of 12 counts each. Place disposable liners in it.

Add almonds, swerve, orange zest, oil, vanilla and salt into the food processor. Process until smooth.

Divide equally into 2 bowls. Add cocoa powder into one of the bowls and mix well.

Spoon vanilla mixture in one half of the muffin cup and immediately fill the remaining half portion with cocoa mixture. Tap the muffin tin on your countertop lightly for the mixture to settle.

Place in the freezer until firm. Remove from the freezer and remove from the muffin tin.

Transfer into an airtight container and refrigerate until use. It can last for 5 days.

Fudgy Macadamia Chocolate Fat Bombs

Serves: 12

Ingredients:

4 ounces cocoa butter

4 tablespoons swerve

½ cup heavy cream or coconut oil

4 tablespoons cocoa powder, unsweetened

8 ounces macadamia nuts, chopped

Directions:

Add cocoa butter into a heatproof bowl. Place the bowl in a double boiler until the cocoa butter melts. Stir occasionally. Remove the bowl from the double boiler.

Add cocoa powder and swerve and mix well.

Add macadamia nuts and mix well. Divide the mixture into 12 fat bomb molds or paper candy cups. Cool completely.

Refrigerate until firm.

Remove from the refrigerator about 30 minutes before serving.

Creamsicle Fat Bombs

Serves: 20

Ingredients:

1 cup coconut oil

8 ounces cream cheese

20 drops liquid stevia or to taste

1 cup heavy whipping cream

2 teaspoons orange vanilla mio

Directions:

Add coconut oil, cream cheese, stevia, whipping cream and orange vanilla mio into a bowl. Blend until smooth using an immersion blender. Just in case the ingredients are not blending well, then microwave on high for 20 seconds to soften.

Pour into silicone tray or fat bomb molds. Freeze

for a couple of hours or until firm.

Remove from the mold and serve. Store the remaining fat bombs in an airtight container. This can be refrigerated until further use.

Ketogenic Lunch Recipes

Cream of Chicken Soup without Cream

Serves: 4

Ingredients:

2 medium cauliflowers, cut into florets

2 cups chicken broth

1 teaspoon sea salt

Freshly ground pepper to taste

¼ teaspoon dried thyme

½ cup cooked, finely chopped chicken thighs

1 1/3 cups almond milk, unsweetened

2 teaspoons onion powder

½ teaspoon garlic powder

¼ teaspoon celery seeds (optional)

½ cup Collagen protein beef gelatin (optional)

Directions:

Add cauliflower, broth, salt, pepper, thyme, milk, onion powder, garlic powder and celery seeds into a soup pot.

Place the soup pot over medium heat. Cover with a lid.

When it boils, lower heat and simmer until cauliflower is soft.

Turn off the heat. Take out about a cup of the cooked liquid and add into a bowl.

Add a teaspoon of gelatin at a time into the bowl of cooked liquid. Whisk well each time until the gelatin is dissolved. Continue doing this until the entire gelatin is added.

Pour the gelatin mixture into a blender. Also add the cooked cauliflower mixture.

Blend until smooth and creamy.

Pour the soup back into the pot. Place the pot over low heat.

Add chicken and stir. Cover and heat thoroughly.

Ladle into soup bowls and serve.

Asparagus & Sorrel Bisque

Serves: 4

Ingredients:

1 tablespoon unsalted butter

1 large leek, thinly sliced

½ teaspoon kosher salt or to taste

Pepper to taste

1 pound asparagus, trimmed

¼ cup crème Fraiche

1 tablespoon extra-virgin olive oil

1 stalk green garlic, sliced

2 cups low sodium vegetable broth

2 cups sorrel or baby arugula + extra to garnish

1 radish, sliced, to garnish

Directions:

Place a soup pot over medium heat. Add oil and butter. When butter melts, add leeks, green garlic and asparagus and stir for a minute.

Add salt, pepper and broth.

Cover and cook until asparagus is tender. Turn off the heat.

Cool completely.

Pour soup into a bowl and keep in the refrigerator for 2-3 hours. Do not cover the bowl.

Remove the chilled soup from the refrigerator and transfer into a blender.

Add sorrel and blend for 40 to 50 seconds or until smooth.

Taste and adjust the seasoning if required.

Ladle into soup bowls. Sprinkle some pepper on top. Top with a tablespoon of crème Fraiche in each bowl.

Place radish slices on top and serve.

Avocado Cucumber Gazpacho

Serves: 3

Ingredients:

1 medium cucumber, peeled, deseeded, chopped

½ jalapeño, deseeded, chopped

1 medium avocado, peeled, pitted, chopped

2 tablespoons apple cider vinegar

½ teaspoon salt or to taste

Pepper to taste

A handful fresh cilantro or basil, chopped

1 clove garlic, peeled, chopped

Directions:

Add cucumber, jalapeño, avocado, cilantro, vinegar, salt, pepper and garlic into a blender and blend for 30-40 seconds.

Add water and blend until smooth.

Taste and adjust the seasoning if required.

Pour into a bowl. Cover and refrigerate until use.

Ladle into soup bowls and serve.

Green Lemon Smoothie

Serves: 2

Ingredients:

1 large avocado, peeled, pitted, chopped

6 tablespoons lemon juice

1 cup coconut milk or coconut cream

2 scoops bulletproof collagen protein

2 cups ice cubes

1 cucumber, chopped

4 cups fresh spinach, chopped

2 tablespoons brain octane oil

2 scoops bulletproof whey protein

Xylitol or stevia to taste

5-6 drops lemon essential oil

Optional toppings:

Nut butter or seed butter of your choice

A handful raspberries or blueberries

2 tablespoons shredded coconut

Grated ginger

Directions:

Lightly steam the spinach leaves. Cool completely. Add avocado, lemon juice, coconut milk, ice cubes, cucumber, spinach, brain octane oil, stevia and lemon oil into a blender and blend until smooth. Add more water if you prefer a smoothie of thinner consistency.

Add whey protein powder and collagen protein and give short pulses until well incorporated.

Pour into glasses and serve with optional toppings.

Coleslaw-Stuffed Wraps

Serves: 2 (4 wraps each)

Ingredients:

For the coleslaw:

1 ½ cups red cabbage, thinly sliced

6 tablespoons keto-friendly mayonnaise

A pinch salt or to taste

1 green onion, chopped

1 teaspoon apple cider vinegar

Other ingredients:

8 collard leaves, discard stems

3 tablespoons packed alfalfa sprouts

½ pound ground meat of your choice, cooked, chilled

Directions:

To make coleslaw: Add cabbage, mayonnaise, salt,

green onion and vinegar into a bowl and mix well.

To make wraps: Place collard leaves on your countertop.

Place a spoonful of the coleslaw on the edge of each of the leaves, opposite the stem part.

Tuck the sides and roll the leaves. Fasten with toothpicks.

Serve.

Cuban Chayote Salad

Serves: 3

Ingredients:

3 chayote's, peeled

Salt to taste

Pepper to taste

¼ teaspoon mustard powder

2 tablespoons extra-virgin olive oil

Directions:

Place a pot filled with water and chayote over medium heat.

Cook until tender. Drain off the water.

Cool for a while. Chop into 1-inch cubes.

Add oil, salt, pepper and mustard into a bowl.

Whisk well and pour over the chayote.

Toss well. Refrigerate for at least an hour.

Serve as it is or over lettuce leaves.

Cobb Salad with Ranch Dressing

Serves: 4

Ingredients:

4 eggs, hardboiled, peeled, chopped

1 rotisserie chicken, chopped

2 avocados, peeled, pitted, chopped

2 tablespoons chopped chives

6 ounces bacon

4 ounces blue cheese

2 tomatoes, chopped

10 ounces iceberg lettuce

Salt to taste

Pepper to taste

For ranch dressing:

6 tablespoons keto-friendly mayonnaise

4 tablespoons water

2 tablespoons ranch seasoning

Salt to taste

Pepper to taste

Directions:

For the dressing: Toss all the dressing ingredients in a bowl and mix well. Keep it aside so that the flavors can come out.

Place a pan over medium flame. Add bacon and cook until it becomes crisp. Remove and place on a plate.

When cool enough to handle, crumble the bacon. Set aside.

To assemble: Spread lettuce leaves on a serving platter. Scatter the rest of the ingredients of salad over the lettuce.

Pour dressing on top. Sprinkle chives and bacon on top and serve.

Blueberry Salad

Serves: 2-3

Ingredients:

20 blueberries or any other berries of your choice

2 large bags salad leaves

4 teaspoons lemon juice

4 tablespoons coconut oil

1 small onion, sliced

4 tablespoons olive oil

2 large chicken breasts, chopped

Salt to taste

Pepper to taste

Directions:

Place a pan over medium flame. Add coconut oil. When cool enough to handle, add chicken, salt and pepper and cook until tender. Turn off the heat and cool completely.

Transfer into a serving bowl. Add onion, blueberries, lemon juice, salad leaves and oil and toss well.

Serve.

Loaded Chicken Salad

Serves: 2

Ingredients:

1 boneless chicken breast half, halved lengthwise

Himalayan pink salt to taste

½ avocado, peeled, pitted, chopped

1 medium tomato, chopped

¼ red onion, chopped

10 basil leaves, chopped

½ tablespoon olive oil

Pepper to taste

1.8 ounces mozzarella balls

½ jar artichoke hearts

3 stalks asparagus, trimmed, chopped into 2-3 inch pieces

2 cups baby spinach

For dressing:

1 tablespoon extra-virgin olive oil

½ teaspoon Dijon mustard

Himalayan pink salt to taste

¾ teaspoon balsamic vinegar

1 small clove garlic, peeled, minced

Pepper to taste

Directions:

Season the chicken with salt and pepper.

Place a cast iron skillet over medium flame. Heat some oil and add chicken and cook for 3 minutes or until it becomes golden brown. Flip and cook both sides until it turns golden brown and is cooked through.

Place asparagus next to the chicken and cook until the asparagus gets soft. Turn off the heat.

To make dressing: Add all the ingredients of dressing into a small jar. Fasten the lid and shake the jar vigorously until well combined. Set aside for about 30 mins for the flavors to set in.

To serve: Place spinach on a serving platter. Top with chicken, artichoke, avocado, onion, mozzarella and basil.

Drizzle dressing on top and serve.

Cucumber Salad

Serves: 4

Ingredients:

1 pound cucumbers, quartered lengthwise and then sliced

4 tablespoons lemon juice

4 tablespoons mayonnaise

Freshly ground pepper to taste

Salt to taste

Directions:

Add lemon juice, mayonnaise, salt and pepper into a bowl and stir.

Add cucumber and stir until well coated with the dressing.

Tuna Fish Salad

Serves: 2

Ingredients:

4 cups mixed greens

½ cup chopped fresh parsley leaves

20 large kalamata olives, pitted

1 avocado, peeled, pitted, diced

2 cans light tuna in water, drained, chopped

2 large tomatoes, diced

½ cup chopped fresh mint leaves,

2 small zucchini, sliced lengthwise

2 green onions, sliced

2 tablespoons extra-virgin olive oil

½ teaspoon Himalayan sea salt or fine sea salt

2 tablespoons balsamic vinegar

Freshly cracked pepper to taste

Directions:

Preheat a cast iron skillet or grill pan. Place zucchini slices on it and grill on both sides. Remove the grilled zucchini and place on your cutting board.

When it's cool enough, chop into bite-sized pieces.

Add zucchini into a large bowl. Add mixed greens, parsley leaves, kalamata olives, avocado, tuna, tomatoes, mint leaves, zucchini, green onions, extra-virgin olive oil, salt, balsamic vinegar and cracked pepper.

Toss well.

Serve right away.

Turkey-Cheddar Roll-Ups

Serves: 2

Ingredients:

6 slices deli turkey

6 slices cheese

Avocado slices

Cucumber slices

Blueberries

Chopped almonds

Directions:

Place turkey slices on a serving platter. Place a slice of cheese on each.

Place avocado, cucumber, blueberries and almonds. Roll the turkey slices and place with the seam side facing down.

Tofu Frittata

Serves: 4-8

Ingredients:

2 tablespoons olive oil

2 zucchinis, chopped

2 packages firm or extra firm tofu

1 cup nondairy milk of your choice

1 teaspoon dried basil

1 teaspoon ground cumin

½ teaspoon red pepper flakes

4 scallions, chopped

1 large red onion, chopped

15-16 crimini mushrooms, chopped

6 tablespoons nutritional yeast

2 tablespoons arrowroot

½ teaspoon turmeric

Salt to taste

Pepper to taste

2 tomatoes, chopped

½ cup chopped kalamata olives

Cooking spray

Directions:

Grease a casserole dish with cooking spray.

Place a large skillet over medium heat. Add oil and heat. Add onion and sauté until translucent.

Stir in zucchini and mushrooms and sauté until tender. Add salt and pepper to taste and stir. Turn off the heat.

Add tofu, nutritional yeast, milk, arrowroot, cumin, turmeric, basil, salt, pepper and red pepper flakes into a blender and blend until creamy.

Pour over the zucchini mixture and stir.

Transfer into the prepared casserole dish.

Scatter tomatoes, olives and scallions on top.

Bake in a preheated oven at 375 ° F for 45-60 minutes or until frittata is set and top is golden brown.

Remove from the oven and cool for a few minutes.

Cut into wedges and serve.

Zucchini Crust Grilled

Serves: 4

Ingredients:

For zucchini crust bread slices:

8 cups shredded zucchini

1 cup shredded mozzarella cheese

2 teaspoons dried oregano

Pepper to taste

2 eggs

½ cup grated parmesan cheese

Salt to taste

For cheese:

2/3 cup grated sharp cheddar cheese

2 tablespoons butter, at room temperature

Directions:

Place rack in the center of the oven. Place a sheet of parchment paper on a baking sheet. Spray some cooking spray over it.

Add zucchini into a microwave safe bowl and cook on high for 6 minutes.

Place the zucchini on a dishcloth. Bring the ends of the dishcloth together and squeeze the zucchini of excess moisture. Squeeze as much as possible.

Add zucchini, mozzarella cheese, egg, Parmesan cheese, oregano and seasoning. Mix well.

Make 8 equal portions of the mixture and place on the prepared baking sheet.

Form squares of the mixture.

Bake in a preheated oven at 375 ° F for 20 minutes or until light golden brown.

Take out the baking sheet from the oven and let the zucchini bread cool completely.

Carefully remove the zucchini bread crust from the parchment paper.

To assemble: Spread butter on one side of the zucchini bread.

Place a nonstick skillet over medium heat. Place zucchini bread on the skillet, with the buttered side facing down.

Sprinkle about 3 tablespoons cheese over it. Cover with another zucchini bread, butter side facing up. Cook until the underside is golden brown.

Flip sides and cook the other side until golden brown.

Repeat steps 10-13 and make the remaining sandwiches.

Spinach Artichoke Chicken Casserole

Serves: 12

Ingredients:

20 ounces artichoke hearts

8 ounces full fat cream cheese

2 cups parmesan cheese, divided

6 cloves garlic, peeled, minced

20 ounces frozen, chopped spinach, drained, squeezed of excess moisture

8 ounces, full fat, keto-friendly mayonnaise

2 cups shredded mozzarella cheese, divided

2 bags chicken tenderloins, thawed, chopped into chunks

Directions:

Place chicken in a large baking dish. Sprinkle salt and pepper over it.

Bake in a preheated oven at 400°F for 15 minutes.

Meanwhile, add spinach, garlic, artichoke, half the cheeses, mayonnaise and cream cheese into a bowl and mix until well combined.

Remove the baking dish from the oven and spread the spinach mixture over the chicken.

Lower temperature to 350°F and bake for another 20 minutes.

Take the baking dish out of the oven and sprinkle the remaining Parmesan cheese and mozzarella cheese on top.

Set the oven to broil mode. Broil for a few minutes until cheese melts.

Serve.

Chicken Club Stuffed Avocados

Serves: 2

Ingredients:

3 ounces grilled, chicken, diced

1 avocado, halved, pitted

2 slices cooked bacon, crumbled

Juice of ½ lime

2 tablespoons mayonnaise

Salt to taste

Pepper to taste

1 small tomato, diced

A handful cilantro, chopped

Directions:

Carefully scoop the avocado but retain the avocado cases.

Add the scooped avocado into a bowl and mash it with a fork.

Add chicken, most of the bacon, 1-tablespoon lime juice, tomato, mayonnaise, half the cilantro, salt and pepper and mix well.

Fill this mixture in the retained avocado cases. Sprinkle remaining bacon and cilantro. Drizzle remaining lime juice on top and serve.

Iceburgers

Serves: 8

Ingredients:

2 large heads iceberg lettuce

2 red onions, cut into round slices

Salt to taste

8 slices cheddar cheese

Ranch dressing, to serve

8 slices bacon

2 pounds ground beef

Freshly ground pepper to taste

2 tomatoes, sliced

Directions:

Cut 16 large rounds from the iceberg lettuce. These are your buns.

Place a large skillet over medium flame. Add bacon and cook until crisp. Remove bacon with a slotted spoon and place on a plate lined with paper towels. Do not discard the fat in the pan.

Place onion slices and cook for 3 minutes. Flip sides and cook for 3 minutes. Remove onions and place on a plate. Discard the fat remaining in the pan.

Make 8 portions of the ground beef and shape into patties. Sprinkle salt and pepper on the burgers and place on the pan. Cook in batches if required.

Cook until the underside is brown. Flip sides and cook the other side until browned and cooked to the desired doneness.

Place a slice of cheese on each burger. Cover the pan for a few minutes so that the cheese melts.

Place one burger on each of 8 iceberg rounds. Place a slice of bacon on each. Place a tomato slice on each. Spoon some ranch dressing.

Cover with the remaining iceberg rounds. Fasten with toothpicks and serve.

Keto Quiche

Serves: 3

Ingredients:

1 ½ tablespoons coconut oil

1 medium bell peppers, chopped

2 cups chopped spinach

6 medium eggs, whisked

2 tablespoons chopped fresh basil

Salt to taste

Pepper to taste

3 slices bacon, diced

1 small onion, diced

1 small tomato, chopped

7-8 olives, sliced

2 cloves garlic, finely chopped

Salt to taste

Pepper to taste

6 tablespoons coconut cream

Directions:

Place a skillet over medium-high flame. Add oil and once it is heated, add bacon and cook until crisp. Take out the bacon and place on a plate lined with paper towels.

Add bell pepper and onion into the same pan and cook until tender.

Stir in the spinach and cook until spinach wilts. Turn off the heat and cool for 15 minutes.

Meanwhile, add eggs into a bowl and beat it well. Add tomatoes, olives, garlic, bacon, basil, coconut cream and spinach mixture. Mix well. Add salt and pepper to taste.

Pour into a baking dish.

Bake in a preheated oven at 350°F for 15 -30 minutes depending on how you like the eggs to be cooked.

Remove from the oven and allow it to cool for a few minutes.

Cut into 3 equal wedges and serve.

Spinach Artichoke Stuffed Peppers

Serves: 2

Ingredients:

2 bell peppers of different colors, halved

Salt to taste

1 cup shredded rotisserie chicken

½ package (from a 10 ounces package) frozen spinach, thawed, drained, chopped

¾ cup shredded mozzarella cheese, divided

2 tablespoons sour cream

1 clove garlic, minced

Extra-virgin olive oil, to drizzle

Freshly ground pepper to taste

½ can artichoke hearts, coarsely chopped ((from a 14 ounces can)

3 ounces cream cheese, softened

¼ cup grated parmesan cheese

2 tablespoons keto-friendly mayonnaise

A handful fresh parsley, chopped, to garnish

Directions:

Place bell peppers on a baking sheet, with the cut side facing up.

Trickle oil over the bell peppers. Sprinkle salt and pepper over it.

Add chicken, spinach, ¼ cup mozzarella cheese, sour cream, garlic, artichoke hearts, cream cheese, Parmesan cheese, mayonnaise, garlic, salt and pepper into a bowl and mix well.

Divide the mixture into 4 equal portions and fill the bell pepper halves with this mixture.

Sprinkle remaining mozzarella cheese over the peppers.

Bake in a preheated oven at 400°F for 15 -30 minutes or until the peppers are cooked to the desired doneness.

Sprinkle parsley on top and serve.

Ketogenic Dinner Recipes

Chicken Enchilada Bowl

Serves: 4

Ingredients:

1 tablespoon coconut oil

6 tablespoons keto-friendly red enchilada sauce

1 small onion, chopped

½ pound skinless, boneless chicken thighs

2 tablespoons water

½ can (from a 4 ounces can) diced green chilies

Toppings:

½ avocado, peeled, pitted, cubed

2 tablespoons chopped pickled jalapeños

1 small tomato, chopped

½ shredded cheese

4 tablespoons sour cream

To serve:

Cauliflower rice

Any other toppings of your choice

Directions:

Place a skillet over medium heat. Add oil. When the oil is heated, add chicken and cook until light brown all over.

Add enchilada sauce, onion, water and green chilies. Mix well.

Lower the heat and cover with a lid. Simmer until chicken is cooked through.

Remove chicken with a slotted spoon and place on your cutting board. When cool enough to handle, chop the chicken.

Add chicken into the skillet. Simmer until thick.

To assemble: Place cauliflower rice in 4 serving bowls.

Divide the chicken among the bowls. Divide the avocado, jalapeño, tomato, cheese and sour cream among the bowls and serve.

Chicken Philly Cheesesteak

Serves: 6

Ingredients:

20 ounces boneless chicken breasts

1 cup chopped onion

1 teaspoon minced garlic

1 cup diced bell pepper

4 teaspoons olive oil

4 tablespoons Worcestershire sauce

6 slices provolone cheese or queso melting cheese

1 teaspoon onion powder

Pepper to taste

1 teaspoon garlic powder

Salt to taste

Directions:

Freeze the chicken for a while. Place chicken on your cutting board and slice into very thin slices.

Add chicken, Worcestershire sauce, salt, pepper, onion powder, garlic powder into a bowl and mix until the chicken is well coated with the mixture.

Place a skillet over medium heat. Add 2 teaspoons oil. When the oil is heated, add chicken and cook until underside is brown. Flip sides and cook the other side until brown.

Remove chicken with a slotted spoon and place on a plate.

Add 2 teaspoons oil into the same skillet. When the oil is heated, add onion, garlic and bell pepper and sauté until onion turns translucent.

Add chicken and mix well. Remove from heat. Place cheese slices all over the chicken.

Cover and set aside for 5 minutes.

Serve hot.

Cheesy Bacon Ranch Chicken

Serves: 2

Ingredients:

2 chicken breasts, skinless, boneless

1 teaspoon ranch seasoning

2 slices thick-cut bacon

Freshly ground pepper to taste

Salt to taste

1 tablespoon chopped chives

¾ cup shredded mozzarella cheese

Directions:

Place a skillet over medium heat. Add bacon and cook until it becomes crisp. Remove and place on a plate lined with paper towels. When cool enough to handle, crumble and set aside.

Retain about a tablespoon of cooked fat from the skillet and discard the rest.

Season the chicken with salt and pepper and place in the pan. Cook until golden brown and cooked through on both sides.

Lower the heat and season with ranch seasoning. Sprinkle mozzarella on top. Cover and cook until cheese melts.

Turn off the heat. Garnish with bacon and chives and serve.

Spicy Sausage and Cabbage Skillet

Serves: 2

Ingredients:

2 spicy Italian chicken sausages, discard casings, chopped

¾ cup shredded purple cabbage

¾ cup green cabbage, shredded

1 tablespoon coconut oil

1 tablespoon chopped fresh cilantro

¼ cup chopped onion

1 slice Colby Jack cheese

Salt to taste

Directions:

Place a large skillet over medium–high heat. Add oil. When the oil melts, add onion and cabbage and sauté until slightly tender.

Add sausages and cook for about 7-8 minutes.

Place cheese slices on top and cover with a lid. Remove from heat. Let it sit for a few minutes for the cheese to melt.

Sprinkle cilantro and serve hot.

Roasted Chicken Stacks

Serves: 4

Ingredients:

4 small chicken breasts or chicken breast cutlets

4 slices prosciutto

1 ½ teaspoons salt or to taste

1 ½ teaspoons Italian herb blend

3 tablespoons avocado oil

1 savoy cabbage, shredded

2 ½ tablespoons coconut flour

Pepper to taste

6-7 tablespoons bone broth

Directions:

Add coconut flour, herbs and seasonings into a plastic bag and shake until well combined.

Place chicken in it and turn the bag around a few times until chicken is well coated.

Grease a baking sheet with oil.

Make 4 heaps of the cabbage on the baking sheet. Season with salt. Trickle some oil on each heap.

Top with a piece of chicken on each heap. Place a slice of prosciutto on each piece of chicken. Pour remaining oil on each heap.

Roast in a preheated oven at 400 ° F for about 30 minutes.

Pour broth all around the heaps in the pan. Roast for 8-10 minutes.

Remove the stacks with a spatula. Remove one

stack at a time and place on serving plates.

Serve hot.

Buffalo Skillet Chicken

Serves: 2

Ingredients:

½ tablespoon extra-virgin olive oil

½ teaspoon garlic powder

Freshly ground pepper to taste

1 clove garlic, peeled, minced

Cayenne pepper to taste

A handful fresh chives, chopped, to garnish

2 boneless chicken breasts

Kosher salt to taste

1 tablespoon butter

½ cup buffalo sauce

4 slices muenster cheese

Directions:

Place a skillet over medium flame. Add oil. When the oil is heated, add garlic and sauté for a few seconds until aromatic. Add buffalo sauce and cayenne pepper and mix well.

When it begins to simmer, add chicken and coat it well with the sauce.

Place 2 slices Muenster cheese on each piece of chicken. Cover the skillet with a lid. Cook for a few minutes until chicken is tender.

Sprinkle chives on top.

Serve over greens of your choice.

Apple Pork Chops

Serves: 2

Ingredients:

1 tablespoon ghee

2 boneless pork chops

1 tablespoon monk fruit sweetener

A pinch ground nutmeg

¼ teaspoon sea salt

1 chayote, peeled, chopped into ½ inch cubes

½ teaspoon ground cinnamon

½ tablespoon apple cider vinegar

Directions:

Place a skillet over medium heat. Add ghee. When ghee melts, add pork chops and sear for 5 minutes. Flip sides and sear for 5 minutes.

Add chayote, cinnamon, vinegar, salt, nutmeg and monk fruit sweetener and stir. Cook until the pork chops are cooked to the desired doneness (medium-rare or medium).

Transfer the pork chops onto a plate. Continue cooking until chayote is cooked through and resembles cooked apples.

Divide the pork chops and mock apples into 2 plates and serve.

Cheesy Bacon Butternut Squash

Serves: 3

Ingredients:

1 pound butternut squash, peeled, cut into 1 inch cubes

1 clove garlic, peeled, minced

Salt to taste

¼ pound bacon, chopped

¼ cup freshly grated parmesan cheese

1 tablespoon olive oil

1 tablespoon chopped thyme

Freshly ground pepper to taste

¾ cup shredded mozzarella cheese

A handful of fresh parsley, to garnish

Directions:

Place butternut squash in a baking dish. Drizzle

oil over it. Sprinkle salt, pepper, garlic and thyme and toss well.

Top with bacon.

Roast in a preheated oven at 425 ° F for about 30 minutes or until tender.

Sprinkle mozzarella cheese and Parmesan cheese on top. Bake until cheese melts.

Remove from the oven and cool for 5 minutes.

Sprinkle parsley on top and serve.

Italian Parmesan Crusted Pork Cutlets

Serves: 3

Ingredients:

3 pork cutlets

¼ cup parmesan cheese, grated

¼ cup Italian dressing

1-2 tablespoons Italian seasoning or to taste

Directions:

Add Italian dressing into a bowl. Add Italian seasonings and stir.

Place cheese in another bowl.

Place a large frying pan on medium heat.

First, dip the cutlets in the Italian dressing. Shake

to drop off excess dressing.

Next dredge in cheese, and place in it the pan. Cook on both sides until brown and cooked to the desired doneness.

Serve hot.

Egg Roll Bowl

Serves: 3

Ingredients:

½ pound ground pork

1 small onion, thinly sliced

½ head cabbage, thinly sliced (thin and long strips)

1 clove garlic, minced

1 green onion, sliced

½ tablespoon sesame oil

1 tablespoon chicken broth or water

½ teaspoon ground ginger

2 tablespoons liquid aminos or soy sauce

Salt to taste

Pepper to taste

Directions:

Place a pan or wok over medium flame. Add pork and cook until brown. Crumble it with a spatula as it cooks.

Add sesame oil into the pan. Mix well with the pork. Add onions and stir. Sauté until the onions are tender.

Add soy sauce, ginger and garlic and stir.

Add cabbage and stir. Add broth and sauté for a couple of minutes.

Add salt and pepper and stir. Remove from heat. Divide into 3 bowls.

Garnish with green onions and stir.

Lamb Kofta Kebabs

Serves: 4

Ingredients:

1 pound ground grass-fed lamb

1 inch fresh turmeric, peeled, grated + extra to garnish

1 cup finely chopped parsley + extra to garnish

½ teaspoon salt or to taste

Directions:

Add lamb, parsley and turmeric into the food processor and process until well combined. Make 8 equal portions.

Take 8 wooden kebab skewers. Shape kebabs around skewers (1 portion per skewer)

Sprinkle salt on the outside of the kebabs.

Place a sheet of foil on a baking sheet. Place a grilling rack on the baking sheet.

Lay the kebabs on the grill.

Grill in a preheated oven for about 20 minutes. Turn the skewers a few times while grilling.

Remove the kebabs from the skewers and place on a plate. Sprinkle turmeric and parsley on top and serve.

Creamy Cauliflower and Ground Beef Skillet

Serves: 2

Ingredients:

1 tablespoon ghee

1 clove garlic, chopped

½ pound lean ground beef

Freshly cracked pepper to taste

¼ cup keto-friendly mayonnaise + 2 tablespoons extra to top

2 tablespoons toasted sunflower seed butter

½ teaspoon fish sauce

2 large eggs

¼ ripe avocado, peeled, diced

½ tablespoon apple cider vinegar

2 tablespoons chopped onions

2 jalapeños peppers, sliced, divided

½ teaspoon Himalayan salt

½ pound grated cauliflower

¼ cup water

½ tablespoon coconut aminos

½ teaspoon ground cumin

A handful of fresh parsley, chopped

Directions:

Place a cast iron skillet or a heavy-bottomed skillet over medium-high heat.

Add ghee. When ghee melts, add onion, garlic and half the jalapeño pepper and sauté for a few minutes until slightly soft.

Stir in beef, pepper and salt and cook until brown. Break it simultaneously as it cooks.

Reduce heat to medium-low. Stir in the cauliflower and sauté for a couple of minutes.

Add mayonnaise, sun butter, water, coconut aminos, and cumin, and fish sauce into a small bowl and whisk well. Pour into the skillet and mix well. Sauté until slightly dry.

Turn off the heat. Make 2 cavities (big enough for an egg to fit in) in the mixture. Crack an egg into each of the cavities. Season with salt and pepper. Sprinkle the remaining jalapeños pepper slices over it.

Transfer the skillet into a preheated oven. Broil for 8-10 minutes until the eggs are cooked to the desired doneness.

Meanwhile, mix together in a bowl, 2 tablespoons mayonnaise and apple cider vinegar. Drizzle over the skillet.

Top with avocado and parsley. Pierce the egg

yolks and serve right away.

Spinach Mozzarella Stuffed Burgers

Serves: 8

Ingredients:

3 pounds ground chuck

Pepper to taste

4 cups firmly packed fresh spinach

4 tablespoons grated parmesan cheese

1 cup shredded mozzarella cheese

2 teaspoons salt or to taste

Directions:

Add beef, salt and pepper into a bowl and mix well. Divide the mixture into 8 equal portions and shape into patties of about ½ inch thickness. Chill for 30 minutes.

Meanwhile, place a saucepan over medium-high

heat. Add spinach and cook until it wilts. Drain off the cooked liquid and set aside to cool.

Squeeze the spinach of excess moisture and place on your cutting board. Chop into smaller pieces and add into a bowl.

Add mozzarella cheese and Parmesan cheese and mix well.

Divide the mixture into 8 equal portions and place one portion in the middle of each of the patties. Bring together the edges and press the edges together to seal. Reshape into patties.

Place a grill pan over medium-high heat. Place the burger on the grill and cook for 5-6 minutes. Flip sides and cook the other side for 5-6 minutes. Alternately, you can grill or broil the burgers. The internal temperature of the cooked burger should be

165 ° F when checked with a meat thermometer.

Serve as it is or with keto-friendly toppings.

Jalapeño Cheddar Stuffed Burgers

Serves: 8

Ingredients:

3 ½ pounds lean turkey or beef

Salt to taste

Pepper to taste

4 ounces cheddar cheese, shredded

2 fresh jalapeños, deseeded if desired, chopped

¼ cup finely minced onion

½ cup cream cheese

½ teaspoon garlic powder

2 tablespoons olive oil

Keto-friendly toppings of your choice

Directions:

Add cream cheese, garlic powder, cheddar cheese and jalapeño into a bowl and stir. Divide into 8 equal portions.

Add the meat you are using, onion, salt and pepper into a bowl and mix well.

Divide the mixture into 8 equal portions. Shape into patties.

Place one portion of the cream cheese mixture in the middle of each of the patties. Bring together the edges and press the edges together to seal. Reshape into patties.

Place a grill pan over medium-high heat. Place the burger on the grill and cook for 5-6 minutes. Flip sides and cook the other side for 5-6 minutes. Alternately you can grill or broil the burgers in an oven. The internal temperature of the cooked burgers should be 165 ° F when checked with a meat thermometer.

Taco Casserole

Serves: 3

Ingredients:

½ tablespoon extra-virgin olive oil

1 pound ground beef

Freshly ground pepper to taste

½ jalapeño, finely chopped, to garnish

1 cup shredded Mexican cheese

½ cup sour cream, to serve (optional)

1 small onion, chopped

Kosher salt to taste

1 tablespoon keto friendly taco seasoning

3 large eggs, lightly beaten

1 tablespoon chopped fresh parsley, to garnish

Directions:

Place a skillet over medium flame. Add oil. When

the oil is heated, add onion and sauté until translucent.

Stir in beef, salt and pepper. Break it simultaneously as it cooks.

Cook until the meat is not pink anymore.

Add jalapeño and taco seasoning and sauté for a minute or so until aromatic.

Turn off the heat. Discard fat in the pan. Let it cool for a while.

Add eggs into a bowl and whisk well. Transfer the meat into the bowl of eggs and mix well.

Transfer into a baking dish. Spread it evenly. Top with cheese.

Bake in a preheated oven at 350 ° F for about 30 minutes or until set.

Drizzle sour cream on top. Sprinkle parsley and jalapeño and serve.

Cheesy Kale Casserole

Serves: 8

Ingredients:

2 pounds lean ground beef

2 teaspoons kosher salt or to taste

2 teaspoons garlic powder

1 teaspoon pepper powder

2 teaspoons onion powder

20 ounces fresh kale, discard hard ribs and stems, chopped

2 teaspoons dried oregano

8 ounces mozzarella, shredded

4 tablespoons olive oil

4 cups keto-friendly marinara sauce

Directions:

Place an ovenproof dish over medium heat. Add

oil. Once the oil is hot, add beef and cook until it is not pink anymore. Break it simultaneously as it cooks.

Add onion powder, garlic powder, salt, pepper and oregano and stir.

Add kale and stir. Cook until it wilts.

Add marinara sauce and heat thoroughly. Add half the mozzarella and stir.

Remove from heat. Sprinkle remaining mozzarella on top.

Set the oven to broiler mode and preheat the oven.

Transfer the dish into the oven. Broil for a couple of minutes, until cheese melts

Remove from the oven. Cool for 5 minutes and serve.

Taco Stuffed Avocados

Serves: 2

Ingredients:

2 ripe avocados, halved, pitted

½ tablespoon extra-virgin olive oil

½ pound ground beef

Salt to taste

1/3 cup shredded Mexican cheese

¼ cup quartered grape tomatoes

Juice of ½ lime

1 small onion, chopped

½ packet taco seasoning

Freshly ground pepper to taste

¼ cup shredded lettuce

Sour cream, to drizzle

Directions:

Scoop out some of the pulp of the avocado and place on your cutting board. You are left with avocado cases. Set them aside.

Chop the scooped avocado and place in a bowl.

Drizzle lime juice over the chopped avocado and set aside.

Place a skillet over medium flame and add some oil. When the oil is hot, add onion and sauté until they get soft.

Stir in the beef, salt, pepper and taco seasoning. Cook until the meat is not pink anymore. Break it simultaneously as it cooks.

Turn off the heat. Discard the fat in the pan.

Stuff this mixture in the avocado cases. Scatter the retained avocado, lettuce, tomato and cheese.

Drizzle sour cream on top and serve.

Lemon Garlic Shrimp and Celeriac "Grits"

Serves: 4

Ingredients:

For lemon garlic shrimp:

20 large shrimp, peeled, deveined

Juice of 2 lemons

6 cloves garlic, minced

1 teaspoon + 2 tablespoons sea salt

A handful fresh parsley + extra to garnish

4 tablespoons pure avocado oil

1 teaspoon smoked paprika

½ teaspoon + ½ teaspoon pepper powder

Lemon wedges to serve

For Celeriac "Grits:

4 medium celeriac, trim the outer brown layer, cubed

2 tablespoons pure avocado oil

½ teaspoon pepper powder

4 cups chicken stock

2 medium onions, chopped

Sea salt or to taste

4 cloves garlic, peeled, minced

Directions:

To make lemon garlic marinade: Add lemon juice, garlic, avocado oil, paprika, 1 teaspoon salt, paprika, parsley and ½ teaspoon pepper into a bowl. Mix well. Cover and set aside for a while for the flavors to set in.

Place a large pot of water with remaining salt over medium heat. Add remaining pepper and stir.

When it begins to boil, add shrimp and cook until shrimp turns pink. Turn off the heat.

Drain and add shrimp into the lemon garlic marinade. Cover with foil and set aside for 10 minutes.

Serve shrimp over celeriac grits. Garnish with parsley and drizzle some lemon juice on top and serve.

To make celeriac "grits": Add the celeriac to the food processor and pulse until you get corn grit like texture.

Place a large nonstick skillet over medium-high heat. Add oil. When the oil is heated, add onions and sauté until translucent. Add garlic and sauté until fragrant.

Add rest of the ingredients into the skillet and stir.

Cover and cook for 10-12 minutes. Uncover and cook until most of the liquid is absorbed.

Serve hot.

Salmon and Creamy Turmeric Veggies

Serves: 2

Ingredients:

2 tablespoons coconut oil or avocado oil

2 small cloves garlic, minced

½ tablespoon grated fresh turmeric

2 tablespoons water

½ tablespoon lime juice

1 ½ cups cauliflower florets

2 wild Alaskan salmon fillets (6 ounces each)

1 small onion, thinly sliced

1 ½ cups broccoli florets

½ tablespoon minced fresh ginger

¼ cup full fat coconut milk

Zest of ½ lemon, grated

Freshly ground pepper to taste

Salt to taste

½ tablespoon lemon juice

Directions:

Place a large cast iron skillet over medium heat. Add oil. When the oil is heated, add onion, ginger, garlic and turmeric and sauté until golden brown in color.

Add water, coconut milk, lemon juice and zest and stir.

When it begins to boil, add vegetables, salt, and pepper, and mix well. Turn off the heat and cover with a lid.

Meanwhile, place a grill pan over medium heat. Let the pan heat.

Sprinkle salt and pepper over the salmon and rub it into it.

Place on the grill and cook for 5 minutes. Flip sides and cook for 5 minutes.

Serve salmon with the cooked vegetables.

Vegan Alfredo

Serves: 8

Ingredients:

1 large head cauliflower, chopped (about 8 cups)

4 cloves garlic, smashed, minced

4 ½ cups almond milk

Juice of a lemon

4 tablespoons olive oil

A handful pine nuts

Salt to taste

Pepper to taste

4 teaspoons dried basil

4 teaspoons dried oregano

½ cup + 2 tablespoons nutritional yeast

Zucchini noodles to serve

Directions:

Place a large pot over medium heat. Add oil. When the oil is heated, add garlic and pine nuts and sauté until garlic turns golden brown in color.

Pour almond milk.

When it begins to boil, lower heat and add cauliflower, salt, pepper and dried herbs and cook until tender.

Turn off the heat and blend with an immersion blender until smooth.

Add nutritional yeast and lemon juice and blend until well combined.

Serve over zucchini noodles or any other keto-friendly noodles of your choice, garnished with basil.

Pizza

Serves: 2

Ingredients:

For pizza crust:

4 large eggs

2 tablespoons psyllium husk powder

Salt to taste

4 tablespoons parmesan cheese

1 teaspoon Italian seasoning

4 teaspoons oil

For toppings:

3 ounces mozzarella cheese, shredded

A handful fresh basil, chopped

6 tablespoons keto-friendly tomato sauce

Directions:

To make the crust: Add eggs, psyllium husk powder into a bowl. Blend with an immersion blender until well combined.

Place a frying pan over medium heat and add oil. When the oil is hot, place half the crust mixture at the center of the pan. Press it lightly, spreading it simultaneously into a round.

Cook until golden brown. Flip sides and cook the other side well too.

Transfer onto a baking sheet.

Repeat the above 3 steps with the remaining crust.

Spread tomato sauce over the crust. Sprinkle cheese on top.

Set the oven to broiler mode. Broil for a couple

of minutes until cheese melts.

Serve.

CONCLUSION

As we come to the end of the book, I would like to thank you again for purchasing it and spending your time in reading through it. I hope you found this book a useful and informative read.

By now, you understand how ketosis works and the keto diet more than you did before you began. You can see why this has gained a cult following over the years. The keto diet will help you lose weight and also reap many other benefits that will help in improving your health and overall well being.

The diet is easy to follow and allows you to enjoy most of the food that other diets would probably ask you to give up. Now you can enjoy that dollop of butter without any guilt. And the best part is, you will know that you are losing weight even while you eat these fatty foods. Follow the list of keto-friendly foods given in the book to ensure you are following the keto diet requirements. Reducing carbs from your diet will play a big role in this.

Use the recipes given here to help you whip up some delicious keto-friendly meals, to begin with. Once you see the keto diet work for you, you may even recommend this keto guide to other friends or family who could use it for themselves.

www.ingramcontent.com/pod-product-compliance
Lightning Source LLC
Chambersburg PA
CBHW020316290526
45785CB00007B/2811
* 9 7 8 1 0 7 9 9 7 1 1 5 6 *